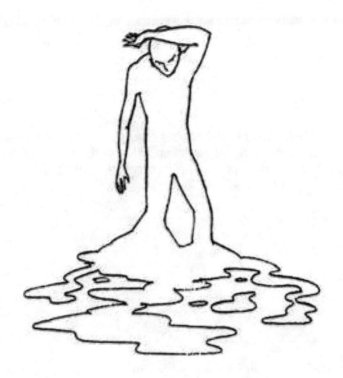

# If You Don't Take Care of Your Body

## of Your Body

### Lifestyle Journal

Information contained in this book should not be used to alter a medically prescribed regimen or as a form of self treatment. Consult a licensed physician before beginning this or any other nutrition progr.

Printed in the United States of America.

ISBN # 978-1-892426-07-9
LMA Publishing
Dr. Jane Pentz
www.lifestylemanagement.com
fax and phone: 800-617-4615

# This Book Belongs To:

Name _____

Street Address _____

City _____ State _____ Zip _____

Phone _____

E-mail _____

Welcome to the beginning of a new life;  a life in which you are in charge of your health.  No more excuses. Today is the first day of taking control.

*"Success in a journey.....Not a destination."*

So stay brave and don't let anything get in your way.

# The Challenge

**I challenge you to a life-changing program. T**his challenge requires dedication and fortitude on your part. I challenge you to make small commitments to yourself and keep them. Begin with small changes; ones that you can live with and are relatively easy to accomplish. Don't set a goal of exercising 30 minutes every day for the next 7 days if you are not exercising at all right now. You will set yourself up to fail, and the whole process will simply reinforce your reactive responses; i.e., I knew I couldn't do it.

Perhaps your goal may be as simple as walking to and from your car parked at the furthermost point in the parking lot. Great! You can then progress to climbing the stairs etc.

Your goal may be to become an active person by walking. Great! You can progress to 10 minutes per day for 3 out of 7 days; and ultimately work towards your goal of walking 10 minutes per day 5 out of 7 days.

Perhaps your goal is to reduce cholesterol levels by limiting your saturated fat intake. Great! Follow the same process. Begin by cutting down on one of your favorite saturated fatty foods, i.e., I'll have a hamburger every other day instead of every day.

# Beginning The Challenge

Start off initially by looking at setting long range goals. Use the following table to organize your thoughts. List two results you wish to accomplish in the next year (always keeping in mind your ultimate goal of achieving and maintaining optimum health).

These goals will need to be occasionally revised and reviewed. Above all, if you feel overwhelmed, take one step at a time. One small step is better than none. One small goal accomplished builds self-esteem and confidence. Many "sincere" large goals failed destroy self-esteem and confidence.

# Long Range Health Goals

Within one year I will:

Goal 1-Exercise: _____

_____

_____

_____

_____

_____

Goal 2- Healthy Eating: _____

_____

_____

_____

_____

Now transform these long range goals into shorter range goals which are still reasonable, measurable, specific, etc. What is it that you wish to accomplish in the next 12 weeks, keeping in mind your long range goals.

Within 12 weeks I will:

Goal 1-Exercise: _____

_____

_____

_____

Goal 2- Healthy Eating: _____

_____

_____

_____

_____

# This Month's Goals

To accomplish my ultimate long range goals, by the end of this month

I will:

Exercise: _____

_____

_____

_____

_____

_____

_____

Healthy Eating: _____

_____

_____

_____

_____

_____

_____

# Living The Challenge

Now that you have identified what it is you will do in the next month, use the following pages to identify your weekly goals and record your daily exercise and eating.

At the end of each week, you can review your journal to see if you have accomplished the tasks you set. While this process is arduous and time consuming it produces the wanted results - you will have become a proactive person in charge of your own health.

# How to use Your Lifestyle Journal:

First, read the agreement on the next page carefully and sign it only if you are ready to *Live the Challenge.*

Second, identify your weekly goals and write them down in your journal.

Third, use the daily weekly pages to record your exercise and eating.

There's no hurry. Success isn't in how much do in the next month. Success is in completing what you say you will do, no matter what it is.

**Good Luck and Don't Give Up! The life you save is your own!** Each commitment you keep is one small step towards taking charge of your health. Remember, mankind needs you to stay healthy so you can share your uniqueness with the world.

# Lifestyle Agreement

## If I Don't Take Care of My Body Where Am I Going to Live?©

Welcome to the rest of My life. I am in charge - no excuses. The next few weeks are crucial to ensuring my success in health and lifelong weight management. I promise to make health my top priority. Many obstacles will undoubtedly crop up, but I will not let them stand in my way. There is nothing more precious than my health.

I am aware that I will probably go through several psychological stages during the next several weeks. I will be looking at what causes me to overeat and/or what prevents me from exercising. Eating issues may well be a cover up for other more deep rooted problems. During these next few weeks I must continuously ask myself if the changes I am making are lifestyle changes - changes that I can live with the rest of my life without feeling deprived or stressed. If these changes are difficult and "unpleasant", then I must "reevaluate". I will work to make these next few weeks the "beginning of the rest of my life".

I will also keep a lifestyle record. Keeping a record can improve my chances of success, and can actually decrease my obsession with food.

I realize that I must do the work. While someone can educate me as to how to Take Care Of My Body, I, alone, am responsible for making the changes.

I _____ will follow the exercise program as set forth in my goals and objectives. I _____ will also make changes in my eating patterns as set forth in my goals and objectives.


Signed: _____ Witness: _____

Date: _____ Date: _____

# Completing Your Journal - Eating

When completing your journal pages, write down the name of the food, the time of day and your mood at the time. This will help in determining if you are eating when stressed, bored, depressed, etc. When completing your journal pages, it is important to estimate how much you are eating. The following chart will help you when estimating how much (or how little) you are eating.

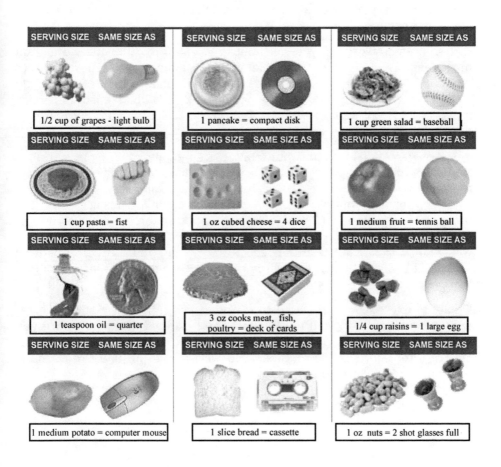

| SERVING SIZE | SAME SIZE AS |
|---|---|
| 1/2 cup of grapes - light bulb | |
| 1 pancake = compact disk | |
| 1 cup green salad = baseball | |
| 1 cup pasta = fist | |
| 1 oz cubed cheese = 4 dice | |
| 1 medium fruit = tennis ball | |
| 1 teaspoon oil = quarter | |
| 3 oz cooks meat, fish, poultry = deck of cards | |
| 1/4 cup raisins = 1 large egg | |
| 1 medium potato = computer mouse | |
| 1 slice bread = cassette | |
| 1 oz nuts = 2 shot glasses full | |

# Completing Your Journal - Exercise

A complete fitness program includes aerobic exercise, resistance training and flexibility. Always check with your physician before beginning an exercise program.

Aerobic exercise (cardiorespiratory) consists of continuous large muscle activities that condition the heart, lungs, and circulatory system. The more aerobically fit you are, the more fat your body will utilize during exercise and at rest. Hence, you will become a more efficient fat burning "machine". The key is to begin slowly.

To become aerobically fit you will want to work up to 30 minutes a day on most days. The intensity of your exercise is also important. You will want to exercise at a comfortable pace; you should be able to talk intermittently while exercising. The Borg scale is designed to help you measure exercise intensity. You will want to work up to 4 on the scale, then up to 7 for short periods of time (see page 14).

Resistance training increases your muscle strength and muscle mass. Unlike fat, which utilizes very few calories, muscle utilizes lots of calories. Hence, the more muscle you have, the higher your metabolic rate (the number of calories your body burns); the younger you are "physiologically"; and the more calories you can eat. You will want to include exercises for every major muscle group (see *If You Don't Take Care of Your Body..*, pages 78-80). You will want to slowly increase the resistance. When you can perform three sets of 8 to 10 repetitions, you will want to increase the resistance by one or two pounds.

Flexibility exercises are required to maintain joint range of motion and reduce the risk of injury and muscle soreness. Always warm up before you stretch. You can warm up by doing aerobic exercise for several minutes, or stretch after your aerobic routine. You will want to include exercises for every major muscle group.

The following is ten tricks to help you stay positive, committed and consistent with your exercise program:

1. Don't work out too hard too fast.  You'll end up sore and uninspired.

2. Schedule your workouts on your calendar as if they're important meetings (which they are!).  Schedule rest days - that will make you want to get back to exercising.

3. Work out in the morning.  You'll get it done and be energized for the rest of the day.

4. Stay off the scales.  Look instead at how well your clothes fit and how good you feel.

5. Choose a role model.  Ask an instructor or a personal trainer for suggestions and advice on how you can reach your goals.

6. Keep a journal.  Chart your progress.

7.  Don't be hard on yourself.  If you miss a workout or a whole week of workouts, simply refocus and make fitness a priority again.

8. Feeling negative?  Just get yourself to do something for 10 minutes.  Most times you will do longer - getting started is the hardest part.

9. Evaluate your progress every three months and alter your workouts to stay motivated.

10. In a rut?  Try working out a different time, try new forms of exercise, or a new piece of equipment, or schedule a few sessions with a personal trainer.

# Lifestyle Journal

Week Number _____     Date _____


By the end of this week I will:

Exercise: _____

_____

_____

_____

_____

_____

_____

_____

Healthy Eating: _____

_____

_____

_____

_____

_____

_____

# Lifestyle Journal

Journal Entry

_____

_____

_____

_____

_____

_____

_____

_____

_____

_____

_____

_____

_____

_____

_____

_____

_____

_____

_____

_____

_____

_____

Week Number: _____     Date: _____     Day: _____

## 1. Cardiovascular Exercise

| Time of Day | Type of Exercise | Number of Minutes | Intensity* |
|---|---|---|---|
| | | | |
| | | | |

## 2. Flexibility/Strengthening Exercise

| Time of Day | Name of Exercise | Number of Times |
|---|---|---|
| | | |
| | | |
| | | |
| | | |
| | | |
| | | |
| | | |
| | | |

## 3. Resistance Exercise

| Time of Day | Name of Exercise | Set # 1 | | Set #2 | | Set # 3 | |
|---|---|---|---|---|---|---|---|
| | | Reps | Weight | Reps | Weight | Reps | Weight |
| | | | | | | | |
| | | | | | | | |
| | | | | | | | |
| | | | | | | | |
| | | | | | | | |
| | | | | | | | |
| | | | | | | | |
| | | | | | | | |
| | | | | | | | |

| * Revised Borg Scale | | Exercise Examples | | |
|---|---|---|---|---|
| 0 nothing at all | 5 strong | 1. Cardiovascular | 2. Flexibility | 3. Resistance |
| .5 very, very weak | 6 | walking, | yoga, Pilates, | free weights, |
| 1 very weak | 7 very strong | jobbing, | muscle | Nautilus eq., |
| 2 weak | 8 | treadmill, | conditioning | Pilaris eq., |
| 3. moderate | 9 | cross trainer, | classes, | Etc. |
| 4. somewhat strong | 10 very very strong, maximal | step class | exercise bands | |

Week Number: _____     Date: _____     Day: _____

## Food Intake Record

| Time of Day | Food Description | Portion Size | Mood* | Calories | Grams | | |
|---|---|---|---|---|---|---|---|
| | | | | | P | F | C |
| | | | | | | | |
| | | | | | | | |
| | | | | | | | |
| | | | | | | | |
| | | | | | | | |
| | | | | | | | |
| | | | | | | | |
| | | | | | | | |
| | | | | | | | |
| | | | | | | | |
| | | | | | | | |
| | | | | | | | |
| | | | | | | | |
| | | | | | | | |
| | | | | | | | |
| | | | | | | | |
| | | | | | | | |
| | | | | | | | |
| | | | | | | | |
| | | | | | | | |
| | | | | | | | |
| | | | | | | | |
| | | | Total | | | | |

---

Number of Servings:

Veggies ☐     Fruits ☐     Calcium ☐

Water ☐     Multivitamin ☐     Other ☐

* Mood Categories:
A = angry
B = bored
C = calm
D = depressed

E = energetic
M = moody
J = joyful

O = overwhelmed
S = stressed
T = tired

Week Number: _____          Date: _____     Day: _____

## 1. Cardiovascular Exercise

| Time of Day | Type of Exercise | Number of Minutes | Intensity* |
|---|---|---|---|
| | | | |
| | | | |

## 2. Flexibility/Strengthening Exercise

| Time of Day | Name of Exercise | Number of Times |
|---|---|---|
| | | |
| | | |
| | | |
| | | |
| | | |
| | | |
| | | |

## 3. Resistance Exercise

| Time of Day | Name of Exercise | Set # 1 | | Set #2 | | Set # 3 | |
|---|---|---|---|---|---|---|---|
| | | Reps | Weight | Reps | Weight | Reps | Weight |
| | | | | | | | |
| | | | | | | | |
| | | | | | | | |
| | | | | | | | |
| | | | | | | | |
| | | | | | | | |
| | | | | | | | |
| | | | | | | | |
| | | | | | | | |

| * Revised Borg Scale | | Exercise Examples | | |
|---|---|---|---|---|
| 0 nothing at all | 5 strong | 1. Cardiovascular | 2. Flexibility | 3. Resistance |
| .5 very, very weak | 6 | walking, | yoga, Pilates, | free weights, |
| 1 very weak | 7 very strong | jobbing, | muscle | Nautilus eq., |
| 2 weak | 8 | treadmill, | conditioning | Pilaris eq., |
| 3. moderate | 9 | cross trainer, | classes, | Etc. |
| 4. somewhat strong | 10 very very strong, maximal | step class | exercise bands | |

Week Number: _____     Date: _____     Day: _____

## Food Intake Record

| Time of Day | Food Description | Portion Size | Mood* | Calories | Grams | | |
|---|---|---|---|---|---|---|---|
| | | | | | P | F | C |
| | | | | | | | |
| | | | | | | | |
| | | | | | | | |
| | | | | | | | |
| | | | | | | | |
| | | | | | | | |
| | | | | | | | |
| | | | | | | | |
| | | | | | | | |
| | | | | | | | |
| | | | | | | | |
| | | | | | | | |
| | | | | | | | |
| | | | | | | | |
| | | | | | | | |
| | | | | | | | |
| | | | | | | | |
| | | | | | | | |
| | | | | | | | |
| | | | | | | | |
| | | | | | | | |
| | | | | | | | |
| | | | Total | | | | |

### Number of Servings:

Veggies [ ]    Fruits [ ]         Calcium [ ]

Water [ ]    Multivitamin [ ]    Other [ ]

* Mood Categories:
A = angry
B = bored
C = calm
D = depressed

E = energetic
M = moody
J = joyful

O = overwhelmed
S = stressed
T = tired

Week Number: _____     Date: _____     Day: _____

## 1. Cardiovascular Exercise

| Time of Day | Type of Exercise | Number of Minutes | Intensity* |
|---|---|---|---|
|  |  |  |  |
|  |  |  |  |

## 2. Flexibility/Strengthening Exercise

| Time of Day | Name of Exercise | Number of Times |
|---|---|---|
|  |  |  |
|  |  |  |
|  |  |  |
|  |  |  |
|  |  |  |
|  |  |  |
|  |  |  |

## 3. Resistance Exercise

| Time of Day | Name of Exercise | Set # 1 | | Set #2 | | Set # 3 | |
|---|---|---|---|---|---|---|---|
|  |  | Reps | Weight | Reps | Weight | Reps | Weight |
|  |  |  |  |  |  |  |  |
|  |  |  |  |  |  |  |  |
|  |  |  |  |  |  |  |  |
|  |  |  |  |  |  |  |  |
|  |  |  |  |  |  |  |  |
|  |  |  |  |  |  |  |  |
|  |  |  |  |  |  |  |  |
|  |  |  |  |  |  |  |  |
|  |  |  |  |  |  |  |  |
|  |  |  |  |  |  |  |  |

| * Revised Borg Scale | Exercise Examples |
|---|---|
| 0 nothing at all     5 strong<br>.5 very, very weak  6<br>1 very weak         7 very strong<br>2 weak               8<br>3. moderate          9<br>4. somewhat strong  10 very very<br>                    strong, maximal | 1. Cardiovascular  2. Flexibility   3. Resistance<br>  walking,          yoga, Pilates,   free weights,<br>  jobbing,          muscle           Nautilus eq.,<br>  treadmill,        conditioning     Pilaris eq.,<br>  cross trainer,    classes,         Etc.<br>  step class        exercise bands |

Week Number: _____     Date: _____     Day: _____

## Food Intake Record

| Time of Day | Food Description | Portion Size | Mood* | Calories | Grams | | |
|---|---|---|---|---|---|---|---|
| | | | | | P | F | C |
| | | | | | | | |
| | | | | | | | |
| | | | | | | | |
| | | | | | | | |
| | | | | | | | |
| | | | | | | | |
| | | | | | | | |
| | | | | | | | |
| | | | | | | | |
| | | | | | | | |
| | | | | | | | |
| | | | | | | | |
| | | | | | | | |
| | | | | | | | |
| | | | | | | | |
| | | | | | | | |
| | | | | | | | |
| | | | | | | | |
| | | | | | | | |
| | | | Total | | | | |

**Number of Servings:**

Veggies [ ]   Fruits [ ]       Calcium [ ]

Water [ ]   Multivitamin [ ]   Other [ ]

* Mood Categories:
A = angry
B = bored
C = calm
D = depressed

E = energetic
M = moody
J = joyful

O = overwhelmed
S = stressed
T = tired

Week Number: _____     Date: _____     Day: _____

## 1. Cardiovascular Exercise

| Time of Day | Type of Exercise | Number of Minutes | Intensity* |
|---|---|---|---|
|  |  |  |  |
|  |  |  |  |

## 2. Flexibility/Strengthening Exercise

| Time of Day | Name of Exercise | Number of Times |
|---|---|---|
|  |  |  |
|  |  |  |
|  |  |  |
|  |  |  |
|  |  |  |
|  |  |  |
|  |  |  |
|  |  |  |

## 3. Resistance Exercise

| Time of Day | Name of Exercise | Set # 1 | | Set #2 | | Set # 3 | |
|---|---|---|---|---|---|---|---|
|  |  | Reps | Weight | Reps | Weight | Reps | Weight |
|  |  |  |  |  |  |  |  |
|  |  |  |  |  |  |  |  |
|  |  |  |  |  |  |  |  |
|  |  |  |  |  |  |  |  |
|  |  |  |  |  |  |  |  |
|  |  |  |  |  |  |  |  |
|  |  |  |  |  |  |  |  |
|  |  |  |  |  |  |  |  |
|  |  |  |  |  |  |  |  |
|  |  |  |  |  |  |  |  |

| * Revised Borg Scale | |
|---|---|
| 0 nothing at all | 5 strong |
| .5 very, very weak | 6 |
| 1 very weak | 7 very strong |
| 2 weak | 8 |
| 3. moderate | 9 |
| 4. somewhat strong | 10 very very strong, maximal |

Exercise Examples

| 1. Cardiovascular | 2. Flexibility | 3. Resistance |
|---|---|---|
| walking, | yoga, Pilates, | free weights, |
| jobbing, | muscle | Nautilus eq., |
| treadmill, | conditioning | Pilaris eq., |
| cross trainer, | classes, | Etc. |
| step class | exercise bands | |

Week Number: _____     Date: _____     Day: _____

## Food Intake Record

| Time of Day | Food Description | Portion Size | Mood* | Calories | Grams P | F | C |
|---|---|---|---|---|---|---|---|
|  |  |  |  |  |  |  |  |
|  |  |  |  |  |  |  |  |
|  |  |  |  |  |  |  |  |
|  |  |  |  |  |  |  |  |
|  |  |  |  |  |  |  |  |
|  |  |  |  |  |  |  |  |
|  |  |  |  |  |  |  |  |
|  |  |  |  |  |  |  |  |
|  |  |  |  |  |  |  |  |
|  |  |  |  |  |  |  |  |
|  |  |  |  |  |  |  |  |
|  |  |  |  |  |  |  |  |
|  |  |  |  |  |  |  |  |
|  |  |  |  |  |  |  |  |
|  |  |  |  |  |  |  |  |
|  |  |  |  |  |  |  |  |
|  |  |  |  |  |  |  |  |
|  |  |  |  |  |  |  |  |
|  |  |  |  |  |  |  |  |
|  |  | Total |  |  |  |  |  |

### Number of Servings:

Veggies [ ]     Fruits [ ]     Calcium [ ]

Water [ ]     Multivitamin [ ]     Other [ ]

* Mood Categories:
A = angry
B = bored
C = calm
D = depressed

E = energetic
M = moody
J = joyful

O = overwhelmed
S = stressed
T = tired

Week Number: _____     Date: _____     Day: _____

## 1. Cardiovascular Exercise

| Time of Day | Type of Exercise | Number of Minutes | Intensity* |
|---|---|---|---|
|  |  |  |  |
|  |  |  |  |

## 2. Flexibility/Strengthening Exercise

| Time of Day | Name of Exercise | Number of Times |
|---|---|---|
|  |  |  |
|  |  |  |
|  |  |  |
|  |  |  |
|  |  |  |
|  |  |  |
|  |  |  |
|  |  |  |

## 3. Resistance Exercise

| Time of Day | Name of Exercise | Set # 1 | | Set #2 | | Set # 3 | |
|---|---|---|---|---|---|---|---|
|  |  | Reps | Weight | Reps | Weight | Reps | Weight |
|  |  |  |  |  |  |  |  |
|  |  |  |  |  |  |  |  |
|  |  |  |  |  |  |  |  |
|  |  |  |  |  |  |  |  |
|  |  |  |  |  |  |  |  |
|  |  |  |  |  |  |  |  |
|  |  |  |  |  |  |  |  |
|  |  |  |  |  |  |  |  |
|  |  |  |  |  |  |  |  |
|  |  |  |  |  |  |  |  |

| * Revised Borg Scale | |
|---|---|
| 0 nothing at all | 5 strong |
| .5 very, very weak | 6 |
| 1 very weak | 7 very strong |
| 2 weak | 8 |
| 3. moderate | 9 |
| 4. somewhat strong | 10 very very strong, maximal |

Exercise Examples

| 1. Cardiovascular | 2. Flexibility | 3. Resistance |
|---|---|---|
| walking, jobbing, treadmill, cross trainer, step class | yoga, Pilates, muscle conditioning classes, exercise bands | free weights, Nautilus eq., Pilaris eq., Etc. |

Week Number: _____     Date: _____     Day: _____

## Food Intake Record

| Time of Day | Food Description | Portion Size | Mood* | Calories | Grams P | F | C |
|---|---|---|---|---|---|---|---|
| | | | | | | | |
| | | | | | | | |
| | | | | | | | |
| | | | | | | | |
| | | | | | | | |
| | | | | | | | |
| | | | | | | | |
| | | | | | | | |
| | | | | | | | |
| | | | | | | | |
| | | | | | | | |
| | | | | | | | |
| | | | | | | | |
| | | | | | | | |
| | | | | | | | |
| | | | | | | | |
| | | | | | | | |
| | | | | | | | |
| | | | | | | | |
| | | | | | | | |
| | | | | | | | |
| | | | | | | | |
| | | | Total | | | | |

### Number of Servings:

Veggies ☐   Fruits ☐   Calcium ☐

Water ☐   Multivitamin ☐   Other ☐

* Mood Categories:
A = angry
B = bored
C = calm
D = depressed

E = energetic
M = moody
J = joyful

O = overwhelmed
S = stressed
T = tired

Week Number: _____     Date: _____     Day: _____

## 1. Cardiovascular Exercise

| Time of Day | Type of Exercise | Number of Minutes | Intensity* |
|---|---|---|---|
| | | | |
| | | | |

## 2. Flexibility/Strengthening Exercise

| Time of Day | Name of Exercise | Number of Times |
|---|---|---|
| | | |
| | | |
| | | |
| | | |
| | | |
| | | |
| | | |
| | | |

## 3. Resistance Exercise

| Time of Day | Name of Exercise | Set # 1 | | Set #2 | | Set # 3 | |
|---|---|---|---|---|---|---|---|
| | | Reps | Weight | Reps | Weight | Reps | Weight |
| | | | | | | | |
| | | | | | | | |
| | | | | | | | |
| | | | | | | | |
| | | | | | | | |
| | | | | | | | |
| | | | | | | | |
| | | | | | | | |
| | | | | | | | |

| * Revised Borg Scale | | Exercise Examples | | |
|---|---|---|---|---|
| 0 nothing at all | 5 strong | 1. Cardiovascular | 2. Flexibility | 3. Resistance |
| .5 very, very weak | 6 | walking, | yoga, Pilates, | free weights, |
| 1 very weak | 7 very strong | jobbing, | muscle | Nautilus eq., |
| 2 weak | 8 | treadmill, | conditioning | Pilaris eq., |
| 3. moderate | 9 | cross trainer, | classes, | Etc. |
| 4. somewhat strong | 10 very very | step class | exercise bands | |
| | strong, maximal | | | |

Week Number: _____     Date: _____     Day: _____

## Food Intake Record

| Time of Day | Food Description | Portion Size | Mood* | Calories | Grams P | F | C |
|---|---|---|---|---|---|---|---|
| | | | | | | | |
| | | | | | | | |
| | | | | | | | |
| | | | | | | | |
| | | | | | | | |
| | | | | | | | |
| | | | | | | | |
| | | | | | | | |
| | | | | | | | |
| | | | | | | | |
| | | | | | | | |
| | | | | | | | |
| | | | | | | | |
| | | | | | | | |
| | | | | | | | |
| | | | | | | | |
| | | | | | | | |
| | | | | | | | |
| | | | | | | | |
| | | | | | | | |
| | | | | | | | |
| | | | | | | | |
| | | | Total | | | | |

### Number of Servings:

Veggies ☐     Fruits ☐         Calcium ☐

Water ☐     Multivitamin ☐     Other ☐

* Mood Categories:
A = angry
B = bored
C = calm
D = depressed

E = energetic
M = moody
J = joyful

O = overwhelmed
S = stressed
T = tired

Week Number: _____     Date: _____   Day: _____

## 1. Cardiovascular Exercise

| Time of Day | Type of Exercise | Number of Minutes | Intensity* |
|---|---|---|---|
|  |  |  |  |
|  |  |  |  |

## 2. Flexibility/Strengthening Exercise

| Time of Day | Name of Exercise | Number of Times |
|---|---|---|
|  |  |  |
|  |  |  |
|  |  |  |
|  |  |  |
|  |  |  |
|  |  |  |
|  |  |  |

## 3. Resistance Exercise

| Time of Day | Name of Exercise | Set # 1 | | Set #2 | | Set # 3 | |
|---|---|---|---|---|---|---|---|
|  |  | Reps | Weight | Reps | Weight | Reps | Weight |
|  |  |  |  |  |  |  |  |
|  |  |  |  |  |  |  |  |
|  |  |  |  |  |  |  |  |
|  |  |  |  |  |  |  |  |
|  |  |  |  |  |  |  |  |
|  |  |  |  |  |  |  |  |
|  |  |  |  |  |  |  |  |
|  |  |  |  |  |  |  |  |
|  |  |  |  |  |  |  |  |
|  |  |  |  |  |  |  |  |

| * Revised Borg Scale | | Exercise Examples | | |
|---|---|---|---|---|
| 0 nothing at all | 5 strong | | | |
| .5 very, very weak | 6 | 1. Cardiovascular | 2. Flexibility | 3. Resistance |
| 1 very weak | 7 very strong | walking, | yoga, Pilates, | free weights, |
| 2 weak | 8 | jobbing, | muscle | Nautilus eq., |
| 3. moderate | 9 | treadmill, | conditioning | Pilaris eq., |
| 4. somewhat strong | 10 very very | cross trainer, | classes, | Etc. |
|  | strong, maximal | step class | exercise bands | |

Week Number: _____     Date: _____     Day: _____

## **Food Intake Record**

| Time of Day | Food Description | Portion Size | Mood* | Calories | Grams | | |
|---|---|---|---|---|---|---|---|
| | | | | | P | F | C |
| | | | | | | | |
| | | | | | | | |
| | | | | | | | |
| | | | | | | | |
| | | | | | | | |
| | | | | | | | |
| | | | | | | | |
| | | | | | | | |
| | | | | | | | |
| | | | | | | | |
| | | | | | | | |
| | | | | | | | |
| | | | | | | | |
| | | | | | | | |
| | | | | | | | |
| | | | | | | | |
| | | | | | | | |
| | | | | | | | |
| | | | | | | | |
| | | | | | | | |
| | | | | | | | |
| | | | | Total | | | |

---

### Number of Servings:

Veggies [ ]    Fruits [ ]       Calcium [ ]

Water [ ]    Multivitamin [ ]    Other [ ]

\* Mood Categories:
A = angry
B = bored
C = calm
D = depressed

E = energetic
M = moody
J = joyful

O = overwhelmed
S = stressed
T = tired

# Lifestyle Journal

Week Number _____    Date _____

By the end of this week I will:

Exercise: _____

_____

_____

_____

_____

_____

_____

_____

Healthy Eating: _____

_____

_____

_____

_____

_____

_____

# Lifestyle Journal

Journal Entry

_____

_____

_____

_____

_____

_____

_____

_____

_____

_____

_____

_____

_____

_____

_____

_____

_____

_____

_____

_____

_____

_____

_____

Week Number: ____    Date: _____    Day: _____

## 1. Cardiovascular Exercise

| Time of Day | Type of Exercise | Number of Minutes | Intensity* |
|---|---|---|---|
| | | | |
| | | | |

## 2. Flexibility/Strengthening Exercise

| Time of Day | Name of Exercise | Number of Times |
|---|---|---|
| | | |
| | | |
| | | |
| | | |
| | | |
| | | |
| | | |
| | | |

## 3. Resistance Exercise

| Time of Day | Name of Exercise | Set # 1 Reps \| Weight | Set #2 Reps \| Weight | Set # 3 Reps \| Weight |
|---|---|---|---|---|
| | | | | |
| | | | | |
| | | | | |
| | | | | |
| | | | | |
| | | | | |
| | | | | |
| | | | | |
| | | | | |
| | | | | |

| * Revised Borg Scale | | Exercise Examples | | |
|---|---|---|---|---|
| 0 nothing at all | 5 strong | 1. Cardiovascular | 2. Flexibility | 3. Resistance |
| .5 very, very weak | 6 | walking, | yoga, Pilates, | free weights, |
| 1 very weak | 7 very strong | jobbing, | muscle | Nautilus eq., |
| 2 weak | 8 | treadmill, | conditioning | Pilaris eq., |
| 3. moderate | 9 | cross trainer, | classes, | Etc. |
| 4. somewhat strong | 10 very very strong, maximal | step class | exercise bands | |

Week Number: _____     Date: _____     Day: _____

## Food Intake Record

| Time of Day | Food Description | Portion Size | Mood* | Calories | Grams | | |
|---|---|---|---|---|---|---|---|
| | | | | | P | F | C |
| | | | | | | | |
| | | | | | | | |
| | | | | | | | |
| | | | | | | | |
| | | | | | | | |
| | | | | | | | |
| | | | | | | | |
| | | | | | | | |
| | | | | | | | |
| | | | | | | | |
| | | | | | | | |
| | | | | | | | |
| | | | | | | | |
| | | | | | | | |
| | | | | | | | |
| | | | | | | | |
| | | | | | | | |
| | | | | | | | |
| | | | | | | | |
| | | | | | | | |
| | | | | | | | |
| | | | | Total | | | |

---

### Number of Servings:

Veggies [ ]     Fruits [ ]     Calcium [ ]

Water [ ]     Multivitamin [ ]     Other [ ]

* Mood Categories:
A = angry
B = bored
C = calm
D = depressed

E = energetic
M = moody
J = joyful

O = overwhelmed
S = stressed
T = tired

Week Number: _____     Date: _____     Day: _____

## 1. Cardiovascular Exercise

| Time of Day | Type of Exercise | Number of Minutes | Intensity* |
|---|---|---|---|
|  |  |  |  |
|  |  |  |  |
|  |  |  |  |

## 2. Flexibility/Strengthening Exercise

| Time of Day | Name of Exercise | Number of Times |
|---|---|---|
|  |  |  |
|  |  |  |
|  |  |  |
|  |  |  |
|  |  |  |
|  |  |  |
|  |  |  |
|  |  |  |

## 3. Resistance Exercise

| Time of Day | Name of Exercise | Set # 1 | | Set #2 | | Set # 3 | |
|---|---|---|---|---|---|---|---|
|  |  | Reps | Weight | Reps | Weight | Reps | Weight |
|  |  |  |  |  |  |  |  |
|  |  |  |  |  |  |  |  |
|  |  |  |  |  |  |  |  |
|  |  |  |  |  |  |  |  |
|  |  |  |  |  |  |  |  |
|  |  |  |  |  |  |  |  |
|  |  |  |  |  |  |  |  |
|  |  |  |  |  |  |  |  |
|  |  |  |  |  |  |  |  |
|  |  |  |  |  |  |  |  |

| * Revised Borg Scale | | Exercise Examples | | |
|---|---|---|---|---|
| 0 nothing at all | 5 strong | 1. Cardiovascular | 2. Flexibility | 3. Resistance |
| .5 very, very weak | 6 | walking, | yoga, Pilates, | free weights, |
| 1 very weak | 7 very strong | jobbing, | muscle | Nautilus eq., |
| 2 weak | 8 | treadmill, | conditioning | Pilaris eq., |
| 3. moderate | 9 | cross trainer, | classes, | Etc. |
| 4. somewhat strong | 10 very very | step class | exercise bands | |
| | strong, maximal | | | |

Week Number: _____     Date: _____     Day: _____

## Food Intake Record

| Time of Day | Food Description | Portion Size | Mood* | Calories | Grams P | F | C |
|---|---|---|---|---|---|---|---|
| | | | | | | | |
| | | | | | | | |
| | | | | | | | |
| | | | | | | | |
| | | | | | | | |
| | | | | | | | |
| | | | | | | | |
| | | | | | | | |
| | | | | | | | |
| | | | | | | | |
| | | | | | | | |
| | | | | | | | |
| | | | | | | | |
| | | | | | | | |
| | | | | | | | |
| | | | | | | | |
| | | | | | | | |
| | | | | | | | |
| | | | | | | | |
| | | | | | | | |
| | | | | | | | |
| | | | | | | | |
| | | | | | | | |
| | | Total | | | | | |

### Number of Servings:

Veggies ☐   Fruits ☐   Calcium ☐

Water ☐   Multivitamin ☐   Other ☐

* Mood Categories:
A = angry
B = bored
C = calm
D = depressed

E = energetic
M = moody
J = joyful

O = overwhelmed
S = stressed
T = tired

Week Number: _____  Date: _____  Day: _____

## 1. Cardiovascular Exercise

| Time of Day | Type of Exercise | Number of Minutes | Intensity* |
|---|---|---|---|
|  |  |  |  |
|  |  |  |  |

## 2. Flexibility/Strengthening Exercise

| Time of Day | Name of Exercise | Number of Times |
|---|---|---|
|  |  |  |
|  |  |  |
|  |  |  |
|  |  |  |
|  |  |  |
|  |  |  |
|  |  |  |
|  |  |  |

## 3. Resistance Exercise

| Time of Day | Name of Exercise | Set # 1 | | Set #2 | | Set # 3 | |
|---|---|---|---|---|---|---|---|
|  |  | Reps | Weight | Reps | Weight | Reps | Weight |
|  |  |  |  |  |  |  |  |
|  |  |  |  |  |  |  |  |
|  |  |  |  |  |  |  |  |
|  |  |  |  |  |  |  |  |
|  |  |  |  |  |  |  |  |
|  |  |  |  |  |  |  |  |
|  |  |  |  |  |  |  |  |
|  |  |  |  |  |  |  |  |
|  |  |  |  |  |  |  |  |
|  |  |  |  |  |  |  |  |

| * Revised Borg Scale | | Exercise Examples | | |
|---|---|---|---|---|
| 0 nothing at all | 5 strong | 1. Cardiovascular | 2. Flexibility | 3. Resistance |
| .5 very, very weak | 6 | walking, | yoga, Pilates, | free weights, |
| 1 very weak | 7 very strong | jobbing, | muscle | Nautilus eq., |
| 2 weak | 8 | treadmill, | conditioning | Pilaris eq., |
| 3. moderate | 9 | cross trainer, | classes, | Etc. |
| 4. somewhat strong | 10 very very | step class | exercise bands | |
| | strong, maximal | | | |

34

Week Number: _____ Date: _____ Day: _____

## Food Intake Record

| Time of Day | Food Description | Portion Size | Mood* | Calories | Grams P | F | C |
|---|---|---|---|---|---|---|---|
|  |  |  |  |  |  |  |  |
|  |  |  |  |  |  |  |  |
|  |  |  |  |  |  |  |  |
|  |  |  |  |  |  |  |  |
|  |  |  |  |  |  |  |  |
|  |  |  |  |  |  |  |  |
|  |  |  |  |  |  |  |  |
|  |  |  |  |  |  |  |  |
|  |  |  |  |  |  |  |  |
|  |  |  |  |  |  |  |  |
|  |  |  |  |  |  |  |  |
|  |  |  |  |  |  |  |  |
|  |  |  |  |  |  |  |  |
|  |  |  |  |  |  |  |  |
|  |  |  |  |  |  |  |  |
|  |  |  |  |  |  |  |  |
|  |  |  |  |  |  |  |  |
|  |  |  |  |  |  |  |  |
|  |  |  |  |  |  |  |  |
|  |  | Total |  |  |  |  |  |

**Number of Servings:**

Veggies ☐   Fruits ☐   Calcium ☐

Water ☐   Multivitamin ☐   Other ☐

* Mood Categories:
A = angry
B = bored
C = calm
D = depressed

E = energetic
M = moody
J = joyful

O = overwhelmed
S = stressed
T = tired

Week Number: _____     Date: _____     Day: _____

## 1. Cardiovascular Exercise

| Time of Day | Type of Exercise | Number of Minutes | Intensity* |
|---|---|---|---|
|  |  |  |  |
|  |  |  |  |

## 2. Flexibility/Strengthening Exercise

| Time of Day | Name of Exercise | Number of Times |
|---|---|---|
|  |  |  |
|  |  |  |
|  |  |  |
|  |  |  |
|  |  |  |
|  |  |  |
|  |  |  |
|  |  |  |

## 3. Resistance Exercise

| Time of Day | Name of Exercise | Set # 1 | | Set #2 | | Set # 3 | |
|---|---|---|---|---|---|---|---|
|  |  | Reps | Weight | Reps | Weight | Reps | Weight |
|  |  |  |  |  |  |  |  |
|  |  |  |  |  |  |  |  |
|  |  |  |  |  |  |  |  |
|  |  |  |  |  |  |  |  |
|  |  |  |  |  |  |  |  |
|  |  |  |  |  |  |  |  |
|  |  |  |  |  |  |  |  |
|  |  |  |  |  |  |  |  |
|  |  |  |  |  |  |  |  |
|  |  |  |  |  |  |  |  |

| * Revised Borg Scale | |
|---|---|
| 0 nothing at all | 5 strong |
| .5 very, very weak | 6 |
| 1 very weak | 7 very strong |
| 2 weak | 8 |
| 3. moderate | 9 |
| 4. somewhat strong | 10 very very strong, maximal |

Exercise Examples

| 1. Cardiovascular | 2. Flexibility | 3. Resistance |
|---|---|---|
| walking, | yoga, Pilates, | free weights, |
| jobbing, | muscle | Nautilus eq., |
| treadmill, | conditioning | Pilaris eq., |
| cross trainer, | classes, | Etc. |
| step class | exercise bands | |

Week Number: _____    Date: _____    Day: _____

## Food Intake Record

| Time of Day | Food Description | Portion Size | Mood* | Calories | Grams P | F | C |
|---|---|---|---|---|---|---|---|
| | | | | | | | |
| | | | | | | | |
| | | | | | | | |
| | | | | | | | |
| | | | | | | | |
| | | | | | | | |
| | | | | | | | |
| | | | | | | | |
| | | | | | | | |
| | | | | | | | |
| | | | | | | | |
| | | | | | | | |
| | | | | | | | |
| | | | | | | | |
| | | | | | | | |
| | | | | | | | |
| | | | | | | | |
| | | | | | | | |
| | | | | | | | |
| | | | | | | | |
| | | | | | | | |
| | | | | | | | |
| | | | | | | | |
| | | | Total | | | | |

---

### Number of Servings:

Veggies ☐    Fruits ☐        Calcium ☐

Water ☐    Multivitamin ☐    Other ☐

* Mood Categories:
A = angry
B = bored
C = calm
D = depressed

E = energetic
M = moody
J = joyful

O = overwhelmed
S = stressed
T = tired

Week Number: _____     Date: _____     Day: _____

## 1. Cardiovascular Exercise

| Time of Day | Type of Exercise | Number of Minutes | Intensity* |
|---|---|---|---|
| | | | |
| | | | |

## 2. Flexibility/Strengthening Exercise

| Time of Day | Name of Exercise | Number of Times |
|---|---|---|
| | | |
| | | |
| | | |
| | | |
| | | |
| | | |
| | | |
| | | |

## 3. Resistance Exercise

| Time of Day | Name of Exercise | Set # 1 | | Set #2 | | Set # 3 | |
|---|---|---|---|---|---|---|---|
| | | Reps | Weight | Reps | Weight | Reps | Weight |
| | | | | | | | |
| | | | | | | | |
| | | | | | | | |
| | | | | | | | |
| | | | | | | | |
| | | | | | | | |
| | | | | | | | |
| | | | | | | | |
| | | | | | | | |
| | | | | | | | |
| | | | | | | | |

| * Revised Borg Scale | | Exercise Examples | | |
|---|---|---|---|---|
| 0 nothing at all | 5 strong | 1. Cardiovascular | 2. Flexibility | 3. Resistance |
| .5 very, very weak | 6 | walking, | yoga, Pilates, | free weights, |
| 1 very weak | 7 very strong | jobbing, | muscle | Nautilus eq., |
| 2 weak | 8 | treadmill, | conditioning | Pilaris eq., |
| 3. moderate | 9 | cross trainer, | classes, | Etc. |
| 4. somewhat strong | 10 very very strong, maximal | step class | exercise bands | |

Week Number: _____     Date: _____     Day: _____

## Food Intake Record

| Time of Day | Food Description | Portion Size | Mood* | Calories | Grams P | F | C |
|---|---|---|---|---|---|---|---|
| | | | | | | | |
| | | | | | | | |
| | | | | | | | |
| | | | | | | | |
| | | | | | | | |
| | | | | | | | |
| | | | | | | | |
| | | | | | | | |
| | | | | | | | |
| | | | | | | | |
| | | | | | | | |
| | | | | | | | |
| | | | | | | | |
| | | | | | | | |
| | | | | | | | |
| | | | | | | | |
| | | | | | | | |
| | | | | | | | |
| | | | | | | | |
| | | | | | | | |
| | | | | | | | |
| | | | | | | | |
| | | | | Total | | | |

Number of Servings:

Veggies [  ]    Fruits [  ]    Calcium [  ]

Water [  ]    Multivitamin [  ]    Other [  ]

* Mood Categories:
A = angry
B = bored
C = calm
D = depressed

E = energetic
M = moody
J = joyful

O = overwhelmed
S = stressed
T = tired

Week Number: _____     Date: _____     Day: _____

## 1. Cardiovascular Exercise

| Time of Day | Type of Exercise | Number of Minutes | Intensity* |
|---|---|---|---|
|  |  |  |  |
|  |  |  |  |

## 2. Flexibility/Strengthening Exercise

| Time of Day | Name of Exercise | Number of Times |
|---|---|---|
|  |  |  |
|  |  |  |
|  |  |  |
|  |  |  |
|  |  |  |
|  |  |  |
|  |  |  |
|  |  |  |

## 3. Resistance Exercise

| Time of Day | Name of Exercise | Set # 1 | | Set #2 | | Set # 3 | |
|---|---|---|---|---|---|---|---|
|  |  | Reps | Weight | Reps | Weight | Reps | Weight |
|  |  |  |  |  |  |  |  |
|  |  |  |  |  |  |  |  |
|  |  |  |  |  |  |  |  |
|  |  |  |  |  |  |  |  |
|  |  |  |  |  |  |  |  |
|  |  |  |  |  |  |  |  |
|  |  |  |  |  |  |  |  |
|  |  |  |  |  |  |  |  |
|  |  |  |  |  |  |  |  |

| * Revised Borg Scale | | Exercise Examples | | |
|---|---|---|---|---|
| 0 nothing at all | 5 strong | 1. Cardiovascular | 2. Flexibility | 3. Resistance |
| .5 very, very weak | 6 | walking, | yoga, Pilates, | free weights, |
| 1 very weak | 7 very strong | jobbing, | muscle | Nautilus eq., |
| 2 weak | 8 | treadmill, | conditioning | Pilaris eq., |
| 3. moderate | 9 | cross trainer, | classes, | Etc. |
| 4. somewhat strong | 10 very very strong, maximal | step class | exercise bands | |

Week Number: _____     Date: _____     Day: _____

## Food Intake Record

| Time of Day | Food Description | Portion Size | Mood* | Calories | Grams | | |
|---|---|---|---|---|---|---|---|
| | | | | | P | F | C |
| | | | | | | | |
| | | | | | | | |
| | | | | | | | |
| | | | | | | | |
| | | | | | | | |
| | | | | | | | |
| | | | | | | | |
| | | | | | | | |
| | | | | | | | |
| | | | | | | | |
| | | | | | | | |
| | | | | | | | |
| | | | | | | | |
| | | | | | | | |
| | | | | | | | |
| | | | | | | | |
| | | | | | | | |
| | | | | | | | |
| | | | | | | | |
| | | | | | | | |
| | | | | | | | |
| | | | | | | | |
| | | | Total | | | | |

### Number of Servings:

Veggies [ ]     Fruits [ ]          Calcium [ ]

Water [ ]     Multivitamin [ ]     Other [ ]

* Mood Categories:
A = angry
B = bored
C = calm
D = depressed

E = energetic
M = moody
J = joyful

O = overwhelmed
S = stressed
T = tired

Week Number: _____     Date: _____     Day: _____

## 1. Cardiovascular Exercise

| Time of Day | Type of Exercise | Number of Minutes | Intensity* |
|---|---|---|---|
|  |  |  |  |
|  |  |  |  |
|  |  |  |  |

## 2. Flexibility/Strengthening Exercise

| Time of Day | Name of Exercise | Number of Times |
|---|---|---|
|  |  |  |
|  |  |  |
|  |  |  |
|  |  |  |
|  |  |  |
|  |  |  |
|  |  |  |
|  |  |  |

## 3. Resistance Exercise

| Time of Day | Name of Exercise | Set # 1 | | Set #2 | | Set # 3 | |
|---|---|---|---|---|---|---|---|
|  |  | Reps | Weight | Reps | Weight | Reps | Weight |
|  |  |  |  |  |  |  |  |
|  |  |  |  |  |  |  |  |
|  |  |  |  |  |  |  |  |
|  |  |  |  |  |  |  |  |
|  |  |  |  |  |  |  |  |
|  |  |  |  |  |  |  |  |
|  |  |  |  |  |  |  |  |
|  |  |  |  |  |  |  |  |
|  |  |  |  |  |  |  |  |
|  |  |  |  |  |  |  |  |
|  |  |  |  |  |  |  |  |

| * Revised Borg Scale | |
|---|---|
| 0 nothing at all | 5 strong |
| .5 very, very weak | 6 |
| 1 very weak | 7 very strong |
| 2 weak | 8 |
| 3. moderate | 9 |
| 4. somewhat strong | 10 very very strong, maximal |

Exercise Examples

| 1. Cardiovascular | 2. Flexibility | 3. Resistance |
|---|---|---|
| walking, jobbing, treadmill, cross trainer, step class | yoga, Pilates, muscle conditioning classes, exercise bands | free weights, Nautilus eq., Pilaris eq., Etc. |

Week Number: _____     Date: _____     Day: _____

## Food Intake Record

| Time of Day | Food Description | Portion Size | Mood* | Calories | Grams P | F | C |
|---|---|---|---|---|---|---|---|
| | | | | | | | |
| | | | | | | | |
| | | | | | | | |
| | | | | | | | |
| | | | | | | | |
| | | | | | | | |
| | | | | | | | |
| | | | | | | | |
| | | | | | | | |
| | | | | | | | |
| | | | | | | | |
| | | | | | | | |
| | | | | | | | |
| | | | | | | | |
| | | | | | | | |
| | | | | | | | |
| | | | | | | | |
| | | | | | | | |
| | | | | | | | |
| | | | | | | | |
| | | | | | | | |
| | | | Total | | | | |

### Number of Servings:

Veggies ☐    Fruits ☐        Calcium ☐

Water ☐    Multivitamin ☐    Other ☐

\* Mood Categories:
A = angry
B = bored
C = calm
D = depressed

E = energetic
M = moody
J = joyful

O = overwhelmed
S = stressed
T = tired

# Lifestyle Journal

Week Number _____     Date _____

By the end of this week I will:

Exercise: _____

_____

_____

_____

_____

_____

_____

_____

Healthy Eating: _____

_____

_____

_____

_____

_____

_____

_____

# Lifestyle Journal

Journal Entry

_____

_____

_____

_____

_____

_____

_____

_____

_____

_____

_____

_____

_____

_____

_____

_____

_____

_____

_____

_____

_____

_____

Week Number: _____     Date: _____     Day: _____

## 1. Cardiovascular Exercise

| Time of Day | Type of Exercise | Number of Minutes | Intensity* |
|---|---|---|---|
|  |  |  |  |
|  |  |  |  |

## 2. Flexibility/Strengthening Exercise

| Time of Day | Name of Exercise | Number of Times |
|---|---|---|
|  |  |  |
|  |  |  |
|  |  |  |
|  |  |  |
|  |  |  |
|  |  |  |
|  |  |  |
|  |  |  |

## 3. Resistance Exercise

| Time of Day | Name of Exercise | Set # 1 | | Set #2 | | Set # 3 | |
|---|---|---|---|---|---|---|---|
|  |  | Reps | Weight | Reps | Weight | Reps | Weight |
|  |  |  |  |  |  |  |  |
|  |  |  |  |  |  |  |  |
|  |  |  |  |  |  |  |  |
|  |  |  |  |  |  |  |  |
|  |  |  |  |  |  |  |  |
|  |  |  |  |  |  |  |  |
|  |  |  |  |  |  |  |  |
|  |  |  |  |  |  |  |  |
|  |  |  |  |  |  |  |  |
|  |  |  |  |  |  |  |  |

| * Revised Borg Scale | | Exercise Examples | | |
|---|---|---|---|---|
| 0 nothing at all | 5 strong | 1. Cardiovascular | 2. Flexibility | 3. Resistance |
| .5 very, very weak | 6 | walking, | yoga, Pilates, | free weights, |
| 1 very weak | 7 very strong | jobbing, | muscle | Nautilus eq., |
| 2 weak | 8 | treadmill, | conditioning | Pilaris eq., |
| 3. moderate | 9 | cross trainer, | classes, | Etc. |
| 4. somewhat strong | 10 very very strong, maximal | step class | exercise bands | |

Week Number: _____     Date: _____     Day: _____

## Food Intake Record

| Time of Day | Food Description | Portion Size | Mood* | Calories | Grams | | |
|---|---|---|---|---|---|---|---|
| | | | | | P | F | C |
| | | | | | | | |
| | | | | | | | |
| | | | | | | | |
| | | | | | | | |
| | | | | | | | |
| | | | | | | | |
| | | | | | | | |
| | | | | | | | |
| | | | | | | | |
| | | | | | | | |
| | | | | | | | |
| | | | | | | | |
| | | | | | | | |
| | | | | | | | |
| | | | | | | | |
| | | | | | | | |
| | | | | | | | |
| | | | | | | | |
| | | | | | | | |
| | | | | | | | |
| | | | | | | | |
| | | | | | | | |
| | | | | | | | |
| | | | Total | | | | |

### Number of Servings:

Veggies [   ]   Fruits [   ]        Calcium [   ]

Water [   ]   Multivitamin [   ]   Other [   ]

* Mood Categories:
A = angry
B = bored
C = calm
D = depressed

E = energetic
M = moody
J = joyful

O = overwhelmed
S = stressed
T = tired

Week Number: _____  Date: _____  Day: _____

## 1. Cardiovascular Exercise

| Time of Day | Type of Exercise | Number of Minutes | Intensity* |
|---|---|---|---|
| | | | |
| | | | |

## 2. Flexibility/Strengthening Exercise

| Time of Day | Name of Exercise | Number of Times |
|---|---|---|
| | | |
| | | |
| | | |
| | | |
| | | |
| | | |
| | | |

## 3. Resistance Exercise

| Time of Day | Name of Exercise | Set # 1 | | Set #2 | | Set # 3 | |
|---|---|---|---|---|---|---|---|
| | | Reps | Weight | Reps | Weight | Reps | Weight |
| | | | | | | | |
| | | | | | | | |
| | | | | | | | |
| | | | | | | | |
| | | | | | | | |
| | | | | | | | |
| | | | | | | | |
| | | | | | | | |
| | | | | | | | |

| * Revised Borg Scale | | Exercise Examples | | |
|---|---|---|---|---|
| 0 nothing at all | 5 strong | 1. Cardiovascular | 2. Flexibility | 3. Resistance |
| .5 very, very weak | 6 | walking, | yoga, Pilates, | free weights, |
| 1 very weak | 7 very strong | jobbing, | muscle | Nautilus eq., |
| 2 weak | 8 | treadmill, | conditioning | Pilaris eq., |
| 3. moderate | 9 | cross trainer, | classes, | Etc. |
| 4. somewhat strong | 10 very very strong, maximal | step class | exercise bands | |

Week Number: _____     Date: _____     Day: _____

## Food Intake Record

| Time of Day | Food Description | Portion Size | Mood* | Calories | Grams | | |
|---|---|---|---|---|---|---|---|
| | | | | | P | F | C |
| | | | | | | | |
| | | | | | | | |
| | | | | | | | |
| | | | | | | | |
| | | | | | | | |
| | | | | | | | |
| | | | | | | | |
| | | | | | | | |
| | | | | | | | |
| | | | | | | | |
| | | | | | | | |
| | | | | | | | |
| | | | | | | | |
| | | | | | | | |
| | | | | | | | |
| | | | | | | | |
| | | | | | | | |
| | | | | | | | |
| | | | | | | | |
| | | | | | | | |
| | | | | | | | |
| | | | | | | | |
| | | | Total | | | | |

---

### Number of Servings:

Veggies [ ]     Fruits [ ]     Calcium [ ]

Water [ ]     Multivitamin [ ]     Other [ ]

* Mood Categories:
A = angry
B = bored
C = calm
D = depressed

E = energetic
M = moody
J = joyful

O = overwhelmed
S = stressed
T = tired

Week Number: _____ Date: _____ Day: _____

## 1. Cardiovascular Exercise

| Time of Day | Type of Exercise | Number of Minutes | Intensity* |
|---|---|---|---|
| | | | |
| | | | |

## 2. Flexibility/Strengthening Exercise

| Time of Day | Name of Exercise | Number of Times |
|---|---|---|
| | | |
| | | |
| | | |
| | | |
| | | |
| | | |
| | | |

## 3. Resistance Exercise

| Time of Day | Name of Exercise | Set # 1 | | Set #2 | | Set # 3 | |
|---|---|---|---|---|---|---|---|
| | | Reps | Weight | Reps | Weight | Reps | Weight |
| | | | | | | | |
| | | | | | | | |
| | | | | | | | |
| | | | | | | | |
| | | | | | | | |
| | | | | | | | |
| | | | | | | | |
| | | | | | | | |
| | | | | | | | |

| * Revised Borg Scale | | Exercise Examples | | |
|---|---|---|---|---|
| 0 nothing at all | 5 strong | 1. Cardiovascular | 2. Flexibility | 3. Resistance |
| .5 very, very weak | 6 | walking, | yoga, Pilates, | free weights, |
| 1 very weak | 7 very strong | jobbing, | muscle | Nautilus eq., |
| 2 weak | 8 | treadmill, | conditioning | Pilaris eq., |
| 3. moderate | 9 | cross trainer, | classes, | Etc. |
| 4. somewhat strong | 10 very very strong, maximal | step class | exercise bands | |

Week Number: _____    Date: _____    Day: _____

## Food Intake Record

| Time of Day | Food Description | Portion Size | Mood* | Calories | Grams |  |  |
|---|---|---|---|---|---|---|---|
|  |  |  |  |  | P | F | C |
|  |  |  |  |  |  |  |  |
|  |  |  |  |  |  |  |  |
|  |  |  |  |  |  |  |  |
|  |  |  |  |  |  |  |  |
|  |  |  |  |  |  |  |  |
|  |  |  |  |  |  |  |  |
|  |  |  |  |  |  |  |  |
|  |  |  |  |  |  |  |  |
|  |  |  |  |  |  |  |  |
|  |  |  |  |  |  |  |  |
|  |  |  |  |  |  |  |  |
|  |  |  |  |  |  |  |  |
|  |  |  |  |  |  |  |  |
|  |  |  |  |  |  |  |  |
|  |  |  |  |  |  |  |  |
|  |  |  |  |  |  |  |  |
|  |  |  |  |  |  |  |  |
|  |  |  |  |  |  |  |  |
|  |  |  |  |  |  |  |  |
|  |  |  |  |  |  |  |  |
|  |  |  |  |  |  |  |  |
|  |  |  |  |  |  |  |  |
|  |  | Total |  |  |  |  |  |

### Number of Servings:

Veggies ☐    Fruits ☐    Calcium ☐

Water ☐    Multivitamin ☐    Other ☐

* Mood Categories:
A = angry
B = bored
C = calm
D = depressed

E = energetic
M = moody
J = joyful

O = overwhelmed
S = stressed
T = tired

Week Number: _____ Date: _____ Day: _____

## 1. Cardiovascular Exercise

| Time of Day | Type of Exercise | Number of Minutes | Intensity* |
|---|---|---|---|
| | | | |
| | | | |

## 2. Flexibility/Strengthening Exercise

| Time of Day | Name of Exercise | Number of Times |
|---|---|---|
| | | |
| | | |
| | | |
| | | |
| | | |
| | | |
| | | |
| | | |

## 3. Resistance Exercise

| Time of Day | Name of Exercise | Set # 1 | | Set #2 | | Set # 3 | |
|---|---|---|---|---|---|---|---|
| | | Reps | Weight | Reps | Weight | Reps | Weight |
| | | | | | | | |
| | | | | | | | |
| | | | | | | | |
| | | | | | | | |
| | | | | | | | |
| | | | | | | | |
| | | | | | | | |
| | | | | | | | |
| | | | | | | | |
| | | | | | | | |

| * Revised Borg Scale | Exercise Examples |
|---|---|

| * Revised Borg Scale | | Exercise Examples | | |
|---|---|---|---|---|
| 0 nothing at all | 5 strong | 1. Cardiovascular | 2. Flexibility | 3. Resistance |
| .5 very, very weak | 6 | walking, | yoga, Pilates, | free weights, |
| 1 very weak | 7 very strong | jobbing, | muscle | Nautilus eq., |
| 2 weak | 8 | treadmill, | conditioning | Pilaris eq., |
| 3. moderate | 9 | cross trainer, | classes, | Etc. |
| 4. somewhat strong | 10 very very | step class | exercise bands | |
| | strong, maximal | | | |

Week Number: _____   Date: _____   Day: _____

## Food Intake Record

| Time of Day | Food Description | Portion Size | Mood* | Calories | Grams P | F | C |
|---|---|---|---|---|---|---|---|
| | | | | | | | |
| | | | | | | | |
| | | | | | | | |
| | | | | | | | |
| | | | | | | | |
| | | | | | | | |
| | | | | | | | |
| | | | | | | | |
| | | | | | | | |
| | | | | | | | |
| | | | | | | | |
| | | | | | | | |
| | | | | | | | |
| | | | | | | | |
| | | | | | | | |
| | | | | | | | |
| | | | | | | | |
| | | | | | | | |
| | | | | | | | |
| | | | | | | | |
| | | Total | | | | | |

---

### Number of Servings:

Veggies ☐    Fruits ☐        Calcium ☐

Water ☐    Multivitamin ☐    Other ☐

* Mood Categories:
A = angry
B = bored          E = energetic    O = overwhelmed
C = calm           M = moody        S = stressed
D = depressed      J = joyful       T = tired

Week Number: _____     Date: _____     Day: _____

## 1. Cardiovascular Exercise

| Time of Day | Type of Exercise | Number of Minutes | Intensity* |
|---|---|---|---|
|  |  |  |  |
|  |  |  |  |

## 2. Flexibility/Strengthening Exercise

| Time of Day | Name of Exercise | Number of Times |
|---|---|---|
|  |  |  |
|  |  |  |
|  |  |  |
|  |  |  |
|  |  |  |
|  |  |  |
|  |  |  |

## 3. Resistance Exercise

| Time of Day | Name of Exercise | Set # 1 | | Set #2 | | Set # 3 | |
|---|---|---|---|---|---|---|---|
|  |  | Reps | Weight | Reps | Weight | Reps | Weight |
|  |  |  |  |  |  |  |  |
|  |  |  |  |  |  |  |  |
|  |  |  |  |  |  |  |  |
|  |  |  |  |  |  |  |  |
|  |  |  |  |  |  |  |  |
|  |  |  |  |  |  |  |  |
|  |  |  |  |  |  |  |  |
|  |  |  |  |  |  |  |  |
|  |  |  |  |  |  |  |  |

| * Revised Borg Scale | | Exercise Examples | | |
|---|---|---|---|---|
| 0 nothing at all | 5 strong | 1. Cardiovascular | 2. Flexibility | 3. Resistance |
| .5 very, very weak | 6 | walking, | yoga, Pilates, | free weights, |
| 1 very weak | 7 very strong | jobbing, | muscle | Nautilus eq., |
| 2 weak | 8 | treadmill, | conditioning | Pilaris eq., |
| 3. moderate | 9 | cross trainer, | classes, | Etc. |
| 4. somewhat strong | 10 very very | step class | exercise bands | |
|  | strong, maximal |  |  |  |

Week Number: _____     Date: _____     Day: _____

## Food Intake Record

| Time of Day | Food Description | Portion Size | Mood* | Calories | Grams P | F | C |
|-------------|------------------|--------------|-------|----------|---------|---|---|
|  |  |  |  |  |  |  |  |
|  |  |  |  |  |  |  |  |
|  |  |  |  |  |  |  |  |
|  |  |  |  |  |  |  |  |
|  |  |  |  |  |  |  |  |
|  |  |  |  |  |  |  |  |
|  |  |  |  |  |  |  |  |
|  |  |  |  |  |  |  |  |
|  |  |  |  |  |  |  |  |
|  |  |  |  |  |  |  |  |
|  |  |  |  |  |  |  |  |
|  |  |  |  |  |  |  |  |
|  |  |  |  |  |  |  |  |
|  |  |  |  |  |  |  |  |
|  |  |  |  |  |  |  |  |
|  |  |  |  |  |  |  |  |
|  |  |  |  |  |  |  |  |
|  |  |  |  |  |  |  |  |
|  |  |  |  |  |  |  |  |
|  |  |  |  |  |  |  |  |
|  |  |  |  |  |  |  |  |
|  |  | Total |  |  |  |  |  |

### Number of Servings:

Veggies [  ]   Fruits [  ]        Calcium [  ]

Water [  ]   Multivitamin [  ]   Other [  ]

* Mood Categories:
A = angry
B = bored
C = calm
D = depressed

E = energetic
M = moody
J = joyful

O = overwhelmed
S = stressed
T = tired

Week Number: _____    Date: _____    Day: _____

## 1. Cardiovascular Exercise

| Time of Day | Type of Exercise | Number of Minutes | Intensity* |
|---|---|---|---|
|  |  |  |  |
|  |  |  |  |

## 2. Flexibility/Strengthening Exercise

| Time of Day | Name of Exercise | Number of Times |
|---|---|---|
|  |  |  |
|  |  |  |
|  |  |  |
|  |  |  |
|  |  |  |
|  |  |  |
|  |  |  |
|  |  |  |

## 3. Resistance Exercise

| Time of Day | Name of Exercise | Set # 1 | | Set #2 | | Set # 3 | |
|---|---|---|---|---|---|---|---|
|  |  | Reps | Weight | Reps | Weight | Reps | Weight |
|  |  |  |  |  |  |  |  |
|  |  |  |  |  |  |  |  |
|  |  |  |  |  |  |  |  |
|  |  |  |  |  |  |  |  |
|  |  |  |  |  |  |  |  |
|  |  |  |  |  |  |  |  |
|  |  |  |  |  |  |  |  |
|  |  |  |  |  |  |  |  |
|  |  |  |  |  |  |  |  |
|  |  |  |  |  |  |  |  |

| * Revised Borg Scale | |
|---|---|
| 0 nothing at all | 5 strong |
| .5 very, very weak | 6 |
| 1 very weak | 7 very strong |
| 2 weak | 8 |
| 3. moderate | 9 |
| 4. somewhat strong | 10 very very strong, maximal |

Exercise Examples

| 1. Cardiovascular | 2. Flexibility | 3. Resistance |
|---|---|---|
| walking, | yoga, Pilates, | free weights, |
| jobbing, | muscle | Nautilus eq., |
| treadmill, | conditioning | Pilaris eq., |
| cross trainer, | classes, | Etc. |
| step class | exercise bands | |

Week Number: _____     Date: _____     Day: _____

## Food Intake Record

| Time of Day | Food Description | Portion Size | Mood* | Calories | Grams | | |
|---|---|---|---|---|---|---|---|
| | | | | | P | F | C |
| | | | | | | | |
| | | | | | | | |
| | | | | | | | |
| | | | | | | | |
| | | | | | | | |
| | | | | | | | |
| | | | | | | | |
| | | | | | | | |
| | | | | | | | |
| | | | | | | | |
| | | | | | | | |
| | | | | | | | |
| | | | | | | | |
| | | | | | | | |
| | | | | | | | |
| | | | | | | | |
| | | | | | | | |
| | | | | | | | |
| | | | | | | | |
| | | | | | | | |
| | | | | | | | |
| | | | | | | | |
| | | Total | | | | | |

### Number of Servings:

Veggies ☐    Fruits ☐    Calcium ☐

Water ☐    Multivitamin ☐    Other ☐

* Mood Categories:
A = angry
B = bored
C = calm
D = depressed

E = energetic
M = moody
J = joyful

O = overwhelmed
S = stressed
T = tired

Week Number: _____ Date: _____ Day: _____

## 1. Cardiovascular Exercise

| Time of Day | Type of Exercise | Number of Minutes | Intensity* |
|---|---|---|---|
|  |  |  |  |
|  |  |  |  |

## 2. Flexibility/Strengthening Exercise

| Time of Day | Name of Exercise | Number of Times |
|---|---|---|
|  |  |  |
|  |  |  |
|  |  |  |
|  |  |  |
|  |  |  |
|  |  |  |
|  |  |  |

## 3. Resistance Exercise

| Time of Day | Name of Exercise | Set # 1 Reps | Weight | Set #2 Reps | Weight | Set # 3 Reps | Weight |
|---|---|---|---|---|---|---|---|
|  |  |  |  |  |  |  |  |
|  |  |  |  |  |  |  |  |
|  |  |  |  |  |  |  |  |
|  |  |  |  |  |  |  |  |
|  |  |  |  |  |  |  |  |
|  |  |  |  |  |  |  |  |
|  |  |  |  |  |  |  |  |
|  |  |  |  |  |  |  |  |
|  |  |  |  |  |  |  |  |
|  |  |  |  |  |  |  |  |

| * Revised Borg Scale | | Exercise Examples | | |
|---|---|---|---|---|
| 0 nothing at all | 5 strong | 1. Cardiovascular | 2. Flexibility | 3. Resistance |
| .5 very, very weak | 6 | walking, | yoga, Pilates, | free weights, |
| 1 very weak | 7 very strong | jobbing, | muscle | Nautilus eq., |
| 2 weak | 8 | treadmill, | conditioning | Pilaris eq., |
| 3. moderate | 9 | cross trainer, | classes, | Etc. |
| 4. somewhat strong | 10 very very strong, maximal | step class | exercise bands | |

Week Number: _____     Date: _____     Day: _____

## Food Intake Record

| Time of Day | Food Description | Portion Size | Mood* | Calories | Grams | | |
|---|---|---|---|---|---|---|---|
| | | | | | P | F | C |
| | | | | | | | |
| | | | | | | | |
| | | | | | | | |
| | | | | | | | |
| | | | | | | | |
| | | | | | | | |
| | | | | | | | |
| | | | | | | | |
| | | | | | | | |
| | | | | | | | |
| | | | | | | | |
| | | | | | | | |
| | | | | | | | |
| | | | | | | | |
| | | | | | | | |
| | | | | | | | |
| | | | | | | | |
| | | | | | | | |
| | | | | | | | |
| | | | | | | | |
| | | | | | | | |
| | | | | | | | |
| | | | | | | | |
| | | | Total | | | | |

---

Number of Servings:

Veggies [ ]    Fruits [ ]         Calcium [ ]

Water [ ]    Multivitamin [ ]    Other [ ]

* Mood Categories:
A = angry
B = bored
C = calm
D = depressed

E = energetic
M = moody
J = joyful

O = overwhelmed
S = stressed
T = tired

# Lifestyle Journal

Week Number _____     Date _____

By the end of this week I will:

Exercise: _____

_____

_____

_____

_____

_____

_____

_____

Healthy Eating: _____

_____

_____

_____

_____

_____

_____

# Lifestyle Journal

Journal Entry

Week Number: _____     Date: _____     Day: _____

## 1. Cardiovascular Exercise

| Time of Day | Type of Exercise | Number of Minutes | Intensity* |
|---|---|---|---|
|  |  |  |  |
|  |  |  |  |

## 2. Flexibility/Strengthening Exercise

| Time of Day | Name of Exercise | Number of Times |
|---|---|---|
|  |  |  |
|  |  |  |
|  |  |  |
|  |  |  |
|  |  |  |
|  |  |  |
|  |  |  |

## 3. Resistance Exercise

| Time of Day | Name of Exercise | Set # 1 Reps \| Weight | Set #2 Reps \| Weight | Set # 3 Reps \| Weight |
|---|---|---|---|---|
|  |  |  |  |  |
|  |  |  |  |  |
|  |  |  |  |  |
|  |  |  |  |  |
|  |  |  |  |  |
|  |  |  |  |  |
|  |  |  |  |  |
|  |  |  |  |  |
|  |  |  |  |  |
|  |  |  |  |  |

| * Revised Borg Scale | | Exercise Examples | | |
|---|---|---|---|---|
| 0 nothing at all | 5 strong | 1. Cardiovascular | 2. Flexibility | 3. Resistance |
| .5 very, very weak | 6 | walking, | yoga, Pilates, | free weights, |
| 1 very weak | 7 very strong | jobbing, | muscle | Nautilus eq., |
| 2 weak | 8 | treadmill, | conditioning | Pilaris eq., |
| 3. moderate | 9 | cross trainer, | classes, | Etc. |
| 4. somewhat strong | 10 very very strong, maximal | step class | exercise bands | |

Week Number: _____     Date: _____     Day: _____

## Food Intake Record

| Time of Day | Food Description | Portion Size | Mood* | Calories | Grams P | F | C |
|---|---|---|---|---|---|---|---|
| | | | | | | | |
| | | | | | | | |
| | | | | | | | |
| | | | | | | | |
| | | | | | | | |
| | | | | | | | |
| | | | | | | | |
| | | | | | | | |
| | | | | | | | |
| | | | | | | | |
| | | | | | | | |
| | | | | | | | |
| | | | | | | | |
| | | | | | | | |
| | | | | | | | |
| | | | | | | | |
| | | | | | | | |
| | | | | | | | |
| | | | Total | | | | |

**Number of Servings:**

Veggies [ ]     Fruits [ ]          Calcium [ ]

Water [ ]     Multivitamin [ ]     Other [ ]

* Mood Categories:
A = angry
B = bored          E = energetic     O = overwhelmed
C = calm           M = moody         S = stressed
D = depressed      J = joyful        T = tired

Week Number: _____     Date: _____   Day: _____

## 1. Cardiovascular Exercise

| Time of Day | Type of Exercise | Number of Minutes | Intensity* |
|---|---|---|---|
|  |  |  |  |
|  |  |  |  |

## 2. Flexibility/Strengthening Exercise

| Time of Day | Name of Exercise | Number of Times |
|---|---|---|
|  |  |  |
|  |  |  |
|  |  |  |
|  |  |  |
|  |  |  |
|  |  |  |
|  |  |  |
|  |  |  |

## 3. Resistance Exercise

| Time of Day | Name of Exercise | Set # 1 | | Set #2 | | Set # 3 | |
|---|---|---|---|---|---|---|---|
|  |  | Reps | Weight | Reps | Weight | Reps | Weight |
|  |  |  |  |  |  |  |  |
|  |  |  |  |  |  |  |  |
|  |  |  |  |  |  |  |  |
|  |  |  |  |  |  |  |  |
|  |  |  |  |  |  |  |  |
|  |  |  |  |  |  |  |  |
|  |  |  |  |  |  |  |  |
|  |  |  |  |  |  |  |  |

| * Revised Borg Scale | | Exercise Examples | | |
|---|---|---|---|---|
| 0 nothing at all | 5 strong | 1. Cardiovascular | 2. Flexibility | 3. Resistance |
| .5 very, very weak | 6 | walking, | yoga, Pilates, | free weights, |
| 1 very weak | 7 very strong | jobbing, | muscle | Nautilus eq., |
| 2 weak | 8 | treadmill, | conditioning | Pilaris eq., |
| 3. moderate | 9 | cross trainer, | classes, | Etc. |
| 4. somewhat strong | 10 very very | step class | exercise bands | |
| | strong, maximal | | | |

Week Number: _____     Date: _____     Day: _____

## Food Intake Record

| Time of Day | Food Description | Portion Size | Mood* | Calories | Grams | | |
|---|---|---|---|---|---|---|---|
| | | | | | P | F | C |
| | | | | | | | |
| | | | | | | | |
| | | | | | | | |
| | | | | | | | |
| | | | | | | | |
| | | | | | | | |
| | | | | | | | |
| | | | | | | | |
| | | | | | | | |
| | | | | | | | |
| | | | | | | | |
| | | | | | | | |
| | | | | | | | |
| | | | | | | | |
| | | | | | | | |
| | | | | | | | |
| | | | | | | | |
| | | | | | | | |
| | | | | | | | |
| | | | | | | | |
| | | | Total | | | | |

**Number of Servings:**

Veggies [   ]   Fruits [   ]        Calcium [   ]

Water [   ]    Multivitamin [   ]   Other [   ]

\* Mood Categories:
A = angry
B = bored
C = calm
D = depressed

E = energetic
M = moody
J = joyful

O = overwhelmed
S = stressed
T = tired

Week Number: _____    Date: _____    Day: _____

## 1. Cardiovascular Exercise

| Time of Day | Type of Exercise | Number of Minutes | Intensity* |
|---|---|---|---|
|  |  |  |  |
|  |  |  |  |
|  |  |  |  |

## 2. Flexibility/Strengthening Exercise

| Time of Day | Name of Exercise | Number of Times |
|---|---|---|
|  |  |  |
|  |  |  |
|  |  |  |
|  |  |  |
|  |  |  |
|  |  |  |
|  |  |  |

## 3. Resistance Exercise

| Time of Day | Name of Exercise | Set # 1 | | Set #2 | | Set # 3 | |
|---|---|---|---|---|---|---|---|
|  |  | Reps | Weight | Reps | Weight | Reps | Weight |
|  |  |  |  |  |  |  |  |
|  |  |  |  |  |  |  |  |
|  |  |  |  |  |  |  |  |
|  |  |  |  |  |  |  |  |
|  |  |  |  |  |  |  |  |
|  |  |  |  |  |  |  |  |
|  |  |  |  |  |  |  |  |
|  |  |  |  |  |  |  |  |
|  |  |  |  |  |  |  |  |
|  |  |  |  |  |  |  |  |

| * Revised Borg Scale | |
|---|---|
| 0 nothing at all | 5 strong |
| .5 very, very weak | 6 |
| 1 very weak | 7 very strong |
| 2 weak | 8 |
| 3. moderate | 9 |
| 4. somewhat strong | 10 very very strong, maximal |

Exercise Examples

| 1. Cardiovascular | 2. Flexibility | 3. Resistance |
|---|---|---|
| walking, jobbing, treadmill, cross trainer, step class | yoga, Pilates, muscle conditioning classes, exercise bands | free weights, Nautilus eq., Pilaris eq., Etc. |

Week Number: _____     Date: _____     Day: _____

## Food Intake Record

| Time of Day | Food Description | Portion Size | Mood* | Calories | Grams P | F | C |
|---|---|---|---|---|---|---|---|
| | | | | | | | |
| | | | | | | | |
| | | | | | | | |
| | | | | | | | |
| | | | | | | | |
| | | | | | | | |
| | | | | | | | |
| | | | | | | | |
| | | | | | | | |
| | | | | | | | |
| | | | | | | | |
| | | | | | | | |
| | | | | | | | |
| | | | | | | | |
| | | | | | | | |
| | | | | | | | |
| | | | | | | | |
| | | | | | | | |
| | | | | | | | |
| | | | | | | | |
| | | | | | | | |
| | | | | | | | |
| | | | | | | | |
| | | | Total | | | | |

---

### Number of Servings:

Veggies ☐    Fruits ☐        Calcium ☐

Water ☐    Multivitamin ☐    Other ☐

* Mood Categories:

A = angry
B = bored
C = calm
D = depressed

E = energetic
M = moody
J = joyful

O = overwhelmed
S = stressed
T = tired

Week Number: _____     Date: _____   Day: _____

## 1. Cardiovascular Exercise

| Time of Day | Type of Exercise | Number of Minutes | Intensity* |
|---|---|---|---|
| | | | |
| | | | |
| | | | |

## 2. Flexibility/Strengthening Exercise

| Time of Day | Name of Exercise | Number of Times |
|---|---|---|
| | | |
| | | |
| | | |
| | | |
| | | |
| | | |
| | | |
| | | |

## 3. Resistance Exercise

| Time of Day | Name of Exercise | Set # 1 | | Set #2 | | Set # 3 | |
|---|---|---|---|---|---|---|---|
| | | Reps | Weight | Reps | Weight | Reps | Weight |
| | | | | | | | |
| | | | | | | | |
| | | | | | | | |
| | | | | | | | |
| | | | | | | | |
| | | | | | | | |
| | | | | | | | |
| | | | | | | | |
| | | | | | | | |
| | | | | | | | |
| | | | | | | | |

| * Revised Borg Scale | | Exercise Examples | | |
|---|---|---|---|---|
| 0 nothing at all | 5 strong | 1. Cardiovascular | 2. Flexibility | 3. Resistance |
| .5 very, very weak | 6 | walking, | yoga, Pilates, | free weights, |
| 1 very weak | 7 very strong | jobbing, | muscle | Nautilus eq., |
| 2 weak | 8 | treadmill, | conditioning | Pilaris eq., |
| 3. moderate | 9 | cross trainer, | classes, | Etc. |
| 4. somewhat strong | 10 very very strong, maximal | step class | exercise bands | |

Week Number: _____     Date: _____     Day: _____

## Food Intake Record

| Time of Day | Food Description | Portion Size | Mood* | Calories | Grams P | F | C |
|---|---|---|---|---|---|---|---|
| | | | | | | | |
| | | | | | | | |
| | | | | | | | |
| | | | | | | | |
| | | | | | | | |
| | | | | | | | |
| | | | | | | | |
| | | | | | | | |
| | | | | | | | |
| | | | | | | | |
| | | | | | | | |
| | | | | | | | |
| | | | | | | | |
| | | | | | | | |
| | | | | | | | |
| | | | | | | | |
| | | | | | | | |
| | | | | | | | |
| | | | | | | | |
| | | | | | | | |
| | | | | | | | |
| | | | | | | | |
| | | | | | | | |
| | | | Total | | | | |

### Number of Servings:

Veggies ☐    Fruits ☐        Calcium ☐

Water ☐    Multivitamin ☐    Other ☐

* Mood Categories:
A = angry
B = bored          E = energetic        O = overwhelmed
C = calm           M = moody            S = stressed
D = depressed      J = joyful           T = tired

Week Number: _____     Date: _____     Day: _____

## 1. Cardiovascular Exercise

| Time of Day | Type of Exercise | Number of Minutes | Intensity* |
|---|---|---|---|
| | | | |
| | | | |
| | | | |

## 2. Flexibility/Strengthening Exercise

| Time of Day | Name of Exercise | Number of Times |
|---|---|---|
| | | |
| | | |
| | | |
| | | |
| | | |
| | | |
| | | |
| | | |

## 3. Resistance Exercise

| Time of Day | Name of Exercise | Set # 1 Reps | Weight | Set #2 Reps | Weight | Set # 3 Reps | Weight |
|---|---|---|---|---|---|---|---|
| | | | | | | | |
| | | | | | | | |
| | | | | | | | |
| | | | | | | | |
| | | | | | | | |
| | | | | | | | |
| | | | | | | | |
| | | | | | | | |
| | | | | | | | |
| | | | | | | | |

| * Revised Borg Scale | Exercise Examples |
|---|---|
| 0  nothing at all       5  strong<br>.5  very, very weak   6<br>1   very weak          7  very strong<br>2   weak                 8<br>3.  moderate            9<br>4.  somewhat strong  10 very very<br>                            strong, maximal | 1. Cardiovascular  2. Flexibility      3. Resistance<br>  walking,              yoga, Pilates,    free weights,<br>  jobbing,              muscle             Nautilus eq.,<br>  treadmill,            conditioning      Pilaris eq.,<br>  cross trainer,       classes,            Etc.<br>  step class            exercise bands |

Week Number: _____    Date: _____    Day: _____

## Food Intake Record

| Time of Day | Food Description | Portion Size | Mood* | Calories | Grams P | F | C |
|---|---|---|---|---|---|---|---|
| | | | | | | | |
| | | | | | | | |
| | | | | | | | |
| | | | | | | | |
| | | | | | | | |
| | | | | | | | |
| | | | | | | | |
| | | | | | | | |
| | | | | | | | |
| | | | | | | | |
| | | | | | | | |
| | | | | | | | |
| | | | | | | | |
| | | | | | | | |
| | | | | | | | |
| | | | | | | | |
| | | | | | | | |
| | | | | | | | |
| | | | | | | | |
| | | | | | | | |
| | | | Total | | | | |

---

<u>Number of Servings:</u>

Veggies [ ]    Fruits [ ]        Calcium [ ]

Water [ ]    Multivitamin [ ]    Other [ ]

\* Mood Categories:
A = angry
B = bored          E = energetic      O = overwhelmed
C = calm           M = moody          S = stressed
D = depressed      J = joyful         T = tired

Week Number: _____     Date: _____     Day: _____

## 1. Cardiovascular Exercise

| Time of Day | Type of Exercise | Number of Minutes | Intensity* |
|---|---|---|---|
|  |  |  |  |
|  |  |  |  |
|  |  |  |  |

## 2. Flexibility/Strengthening Exercise

| Time of Day | Name of Exercise | Number of Times |
|---|---|---|
|  |  |  |
|  |  |  |
|  |  |  |
|  |  |  |
|  |  |  |
|  |  |  |
|  |  |  |
|  |  |  |

## 3. Resistance Exercise

| Time of Day | Name of Exercise | Set # 1 | | Set #2 | | Set # 3 | |
|---|---|---|---|---|---|---|---|
|  |  | Reps | Weight | Reps | Weight | Reps | Weight |
|  |  |  |  |  |  |  |  |
|  |  |  |  |  |  |  |  |
|  |  |  |  |  |  |  |  |
|  |  |  |  |  |  |  |  |
|  |  |  |  |  |  |  |  |
|  |  |  |  |  |  |  |  |
|  |  |  |  |  |  |  |  |
|  |  |  |  |  |  |  |  |
|  |  |  |  |  |  |  |  |
|  |  |  |  |  |  |  |  |

| * Revised Borg Scale | |
|---|---|
| 0 nothing at all | 5 strong |
| .5 very, very weak | 6 |
| 1 very weak | 7 very strong |
| 2 weak | 8 |
| 3. moderate | 9 |
| 4. somewhat strong | 10 very very strong, maximal |

Exercise Examples

| 1. Cardiovascular | 2. Flexibility | 3. Resistance |
|---|---|---|
| walking, | yoga, Pilates, | free weights, |
| jobbing, | muscle | Nautilus eq., |
| treadmill, | conditioning | Pilaris eq., |
| cross trainer, | classes, | Etc. |
| step class | exercise bands | |

Week Number: _____     Date: _____     Day: _____

## Food Intake Record

| Time of Day | Food Description | Portion Size | Mood* | Calories | Grams P | F | C |
|---|---|---|---|---|---|---|---|
| | | | | | | | |
| | | | | | | | |
| | | | | | | | |
| | | | | | | | |
| | | | | | | | |
| | | | | | | | |
| | | | | | | | |
| | | | | | | | |
| | | | | | | | |
| | | | | | | | |
| | | | | | | | |
| | | | | | | | |
| | | | | | | | |
| | | | | | | | |
| | | | | | | | |
| | | | | | | | |
| | | | | | | | |
| | | | | | | | |
| | | | | | | | |
| | | | | | | | |
| | | | Total | | | | |

### Number of Servings:

Veggies [  ]   Fruits [  ]      Calcium [  ]

Water [  ]   Multivitamin [  ]   Other [  ]

* Mood Categories:
A = angry
B = bored      E = energetic      O = overwhelmed
C = calm       M = moody          S = stressed
D = depressed  J = joyful         T = tired

Week Number: _____     Date: _____     Day: _____

## 1. Cardiovascular Exercise

| Time of Day | Type of Exercise | Number of Minutes | Intensity* |
|---|---|---|---|
|  |  |  |  |
|  |  |  |  |

## 2. Flexibility/Strengthening Exercise

| Time of Day | Name of Exercise | Number of Times |
|---|---|---|
|  |  |  |
|  |  |  |
|  |  |  |
|  |  |  |
|  |  |  |
|  |  |  |
|  |  |  |
|  |  |  |

## 3. Resistance Exercise

| Time of Day | Name of Exercise | Set # 1 | | Set #2 | | Set # 3 | |
|---|---|---|---|---|---|---|---|
|  |  | Reps | Weight | Reps | Weight | Reps | Weight |
|  |  |  |  |  |  |  |  |
|  |  |  |  |  |  |  |  |
|  |  |  |  |  |  |  |  |
|  |  |  |  |  |  |  |  |
|  |  |  |  |  |  |  |  |
|  |  |  |  |  |  |  |  |
|  |  |  |  |  |  |  |  |
|  |  |  |  |  |  |  |  |
|  |  |  |  |  |  |  |  |
|  |  |  |  |  |  |  |  |

| * Revised Borg Scale | | Exercise Examples | | |
|---|---|---|---|---|
| 0  nothing at all | 5  strong | | | |
| .5  very, very weak | 6 | 1. Cardiovascular | 2. Flexibility | 3. Resistance |
| 1  very weak | 7  very strong | walking, | yoga, Pilates, | free weights, |
| 2  weak | 8 | jobbing, | muscle | Nautilus eq., |
| 3.  moderate | 9 | treadmill, | conditioning | Pilaris eq., |
| 4.  somewhat strong | 10 very very | cross trainer, | classes, | Etc. |
|  | strong, maximal | step class | exercise bands | |

Week Number: _____     Date: _____     Day: _____

## Food Intake Record

| Time of Day | Food Description | Portion Size | Mood* | Calories | Grams | | |
|---|---|---|---|---|---|---|---|
| | | | | | P | F | C |
| | | | | | | | |
| | | | | | | | |
| | | | | | | | |
| | | | | | | | |
| | | | | | | | |
| | | | | | | | |
| | | | | | | | |
| | | | | | | | |
| | | | | | | | |
| | | | | | | | |
| | | | | | | | |
| | | | | | | | |
| | | | | | | | |
| | | | | | | | |
| | | | | | | | |
| | | | | | | | |
| | | | | | | | |
| | | | | | | | |
| | | | | | | | |
| | | | | | | | |
| | | | | | | | |
| | | | | | | | |
| | | | | Total | | | |

### Number of Servings:

Veggies ☐     Fruits ☐          Calcium ☐

Water ☐       Multivitamin ☐    Other ☐

* Mood Categories:
A = angry
B = bored          E = energetic     O = overwhelmed
C = calm           M = moody         S = stressed
D = depressed      J = joyful        T = tired

LaVergne, TN USA
11 June 2010
185791LV00004B/1/P